Addiction Care Navigation in the Bay Area

Addiction Care Navigation in the Bay Area

A Guide to Programs and Professionals

Eli Merritt, M.D.

*Dedicated to Bay Area patients
and families affected by addiction*

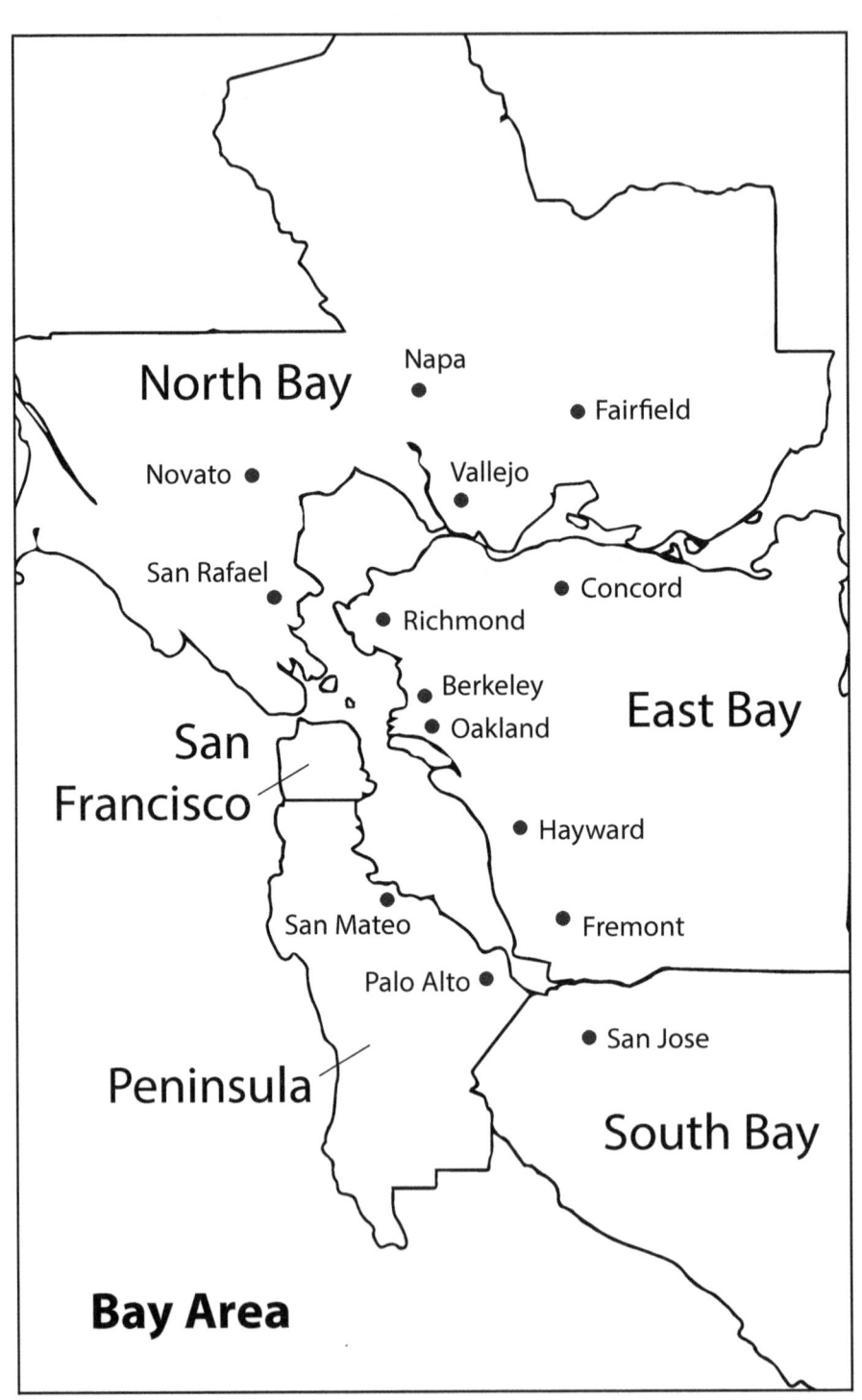

North Bay

Napa

Fairfield

Novato

Vallejo

San Rafael

Concord

Richmond

Berkeley

Oakland

East Bay

San Francisco

Hayward

San Mateo

Fremont

Palo Alto

San Jose

Peninsula

South Bay

Bay Area

Contents

Acknowledgements

In writing the first edition of this book I owe a debt of gratitude to many people. To the expert panelists of the 2017 Addiction Care Navigation in the Bay Area workshop: Howard Kornfeld, M.D.; Rosemary O'Connor, C.P.C.; David Smith, M.D.; and Kristina Wandzilak, C.A.S. To Green Gulch Farm Zen Center. To Tom Comitta, artist and book producer who designed the cover and layout and energized the project from from concept to completion. To Casey Hanley, Care Navigator at Merritt Mental Health, who investigated and compiled resources. To Cynthia Alexander, jack-of-all-trades who energizes Merritt Mental Health daily. And, of course, to my patients and their families who have taught me so much. Thank you.

Preface

We are excited to release this first-of-its-kind Addiction Care Navigation Guide.

Our first hope is that it will serve as a valuable resource for patients, families, health professionals, educators, hospitals, and programs. Our second hope is to expand the guide to include as many addiction-related resources as possible, with the expectation of issuing a second edition in early 2018.

If you are a health professional or program serving individuals with addiction and their families, please contact us to be added to the guide. You can either go to **http://www.merrittmentalhealth. com/addictionguide** and click on "Survey" or reach us at (415) 285-3774 and info@merrittmentalhealth.com.

Introduction

As a psychiatrist who has struggled for more than fifteen years to help patients with addictive disorders, I know firsthand what the challenges are. I know that assessment and diagnosis constitute only the first step, the easiest step. What is far more difficult is knowing who to recommend and where to send patients and families. To which doctors, therapists, interventionists, and family specialists? To what treatment centers, programs, and groups? If you are a health professional, I would be surprised if your experience is different from mine.

In the spirit of confronting this challenge head-on in a collaborative manner, Merritt Mental Health recently organized a conference at Green Gulch Zen Center in Marin called *Addiction Care Navigation in the Bay Area: A Workshop for Health Professionals*. It was not the first workshop I have put on, but it was the best. It was fun, informative, intellectually engaging, and unique.

What made the workshop most unique was not that it was case-based. It was not that that we debated and developed best treatment plans for patients and families. It was that at every step along the way we took out dedicated time to answer a key question: WHO? Specifically WHO does a patient or family member reach out to today for help?

We did not stop at the simple suggestion, "Refer the patient to an addiction specialist." Instead, we generated *specific* Bay Area referrals for every issue and need we encountered during our five hours together. And, post-workshop, we have collected these 50+ referrals into this guide.

What made the workshop unique was the question WHO? What made it excellent was the presence of four addiction experts who shared their extensive expertise and poured out their passion for treatment. They were Howard Kornfeld, M.D., founder and director of Recovery Without Walls; Rosemary O'Connor, C.P.C., founder of ROC Recovery Services; David Smith, M.D., founder of the Haight Ashbury Free Clinics and now medical director of North Bay Recovery Center; and Kristina Wandzilak, C.A.S, interventionist and founder of Full Circle Intervention. I am extremely grateful for the insights, wisdom, and referrals they brought to the table.

In addition to the referrals we generated, we reached many important conclusions about the treatment of addictive disorders. Here I highlight six of the most impactful "pearls of wisdom" we discussed.

Treat the patient and the family, not just the patient. Treating the patient and the family represent the *two fundamental keys* to successful outcomes. Why? Why is a treatment plan for the family essential? The reason is that patterns of interaction between family members and the individual with addiction can either foster or hinder successful treatment of that individual. In their own treatment in Al-Anon or therapy, or work with a family recovery coach or interventionist, family members learn about the disease of addiction, and, vitally, they move every day towards the goals of 1) healthy decision-making and 2) healthy communication with the person suffering addiction. As family members achieve these milestones--healthy decision-making and communication--the effect on the loved one with addiction can be transformative.

Avoid Either/Or thinking. Instead embrace Both/And thinking. The second take-home message from the workshop relates to *how to* treat the person with the addiction. It is rare that a person with addiction does not also have co-occurring grief, depression, anxiety, another mood disorder, or trauma--that is, an underlying mental health condition. We debated extensively whether it is most prudent to start with the treatment of the mental health disorder or the addiction. There was also a second sticky question: Do you treat addiction with AA, psychotherapy, and other psychosocial interventions or with medications and other biological interventions? What was so refreshing and gratifying at the workshop was that we dispensed altogether with Either/Or questions and debates and simply answered, "Yes." We adopted Both/And thinking. Treat addiction *and* anxiety *and* mood disorders. Treat addiction with AA, therapy, *and* medications. Comprehensive, multidisciplinary treatment is categorically the best treatment of all.

Addiction is a treatable disease. The third take-home message, related to the first two, was that addiction is a treatable disease. It can be fatal--we all know that--but we must never lose sight of the truth of successful treatment and recovery. Based on this understanding of addiction, one profound message family members can deliver to the addicted person is: "I love you, and I am not okay losing you to a *treatable disease.*"

Marijuana destroys lives. One of the most surprising conclusions of the workshop, ringing out loud and clear from every corner, was that marijuana destroys lives. There is a fallacy now pervasive in American culture that marijuana, or cannabis, is benign compared to alcohol, opiates, and other substances of abuse. Nothing could be further from the truth. Marijuana is now a more high-potency, addictive, and dangerous substance than ever. Marijuana addiction is not "addiction light." Just blink and it descends rapidly into "addiction heavy." Remarkably, several of our experts

---

"How to Treat Addiction"

Dr. Merritt has summarized the findings of the 2017 Merritt Mental Health workshop in a five-minute video. To watch the video, go to **http://www.merrittmentalhealth.com/addictionguide/**

insisted that marijuana addiction is more difficult to treat than alcohol and opioid addiction.

Good intervention always works. This is a bold claim. On the face of it, since some 20-30% of addicted individuals decline to go into treatment after an intervention, it seems disingenuous or erroneous. However, the claim is in fact 100% correct when seen through the lens of the education and treatment of the family. The reason that good intervention *always* works is that first and foremost intervention is for the family; it is only secondarily a vehicle to get the addicted person into treatment. Intervention educates and sometimes deeply transforms the family. It aids the family to move towards healthy decision-making and healthy communication. Here is the key concept: "The family can get better with or without the addicted person." The family should therefore move forward into maximal health, no matter what the addicted person decides or does.

The key-person approach to treatment. The last take-home message is my favorite. It is the "Key Person Approach to Treating Addiction." At the workshop we often debated the question, "Where does a patient or a family start?" The answer is anywhere, anywhere at all. The reason for this overbroad statement comes back to the essential question of WHO? The question is not where, in fact. It is WHO? Find a key person--that is, a mental health professional with expertise in addiction--and latch on. The person can be a physician, a therapist, an interventionist, a recovery coach, or a sponsor from AA. Just make sure to start with someone who is broad-minded and experienced, and from that pivot point allow the rest of the treatment plan to develop and unfold. Stick with that key person through thick and thin until the patient and the family truly achieve health and wellness.

Addiction is everywhere. Statistics show that it is growing in prevalence, destroying more and more lives every year. Make sure to be on the lookout for it. And, when you see it, ask yourself WHO? Specifically WHO can a patient or family member reach out to today for help?

To aid in this critical pursuit, I have produced this guide. Please make sure to refer patients and family members to it. The guide contains 50+ answers to the vital question WHO?

Additionally, we plan to expand it into a second edition in early 2018. If you are an addiction expert, or an addiction-informed health professional, who works in the Bay Area, please contact us and tell us about the work you do. We would like to include you in the second edition.

The Second Edition of this Guide Will Be Released in Early 2018

If you are a health professional or program with expertise in helping patients and families with addiction, we would like to hear from you. To be included in the guide go to **www. merrittmentalhealth.com/addictionguide** and click on "Survey." You can also call (415) 285-3774 or email info@merrittmentalhealth.com.

1

Interventionists

SAN FRANCISCO

SF Intervention 1-800-868-6173
570 Beale Street #317, San Francisco, CA 94105. http://www.
sfintervention.com. sfintervention@gmail.com. This organization,
founded by Stephen Pfleiderer, specializes in helping adolescents,
adults, and families overcome harmful habits and addictions.
They provide assessments, coaching, interventions, and recovery
workshops.

NORTH BAY

Full Circle Addiction & Recovery Services (415) 747-8224
775 Blithedale Avenue, Mill Valley, CA 94941. http://www.
fullcirclerecoverycenter.net/intervention. This service, founded
by Kristina Wandzilak, endeavors to re-establish the connection
between the family member suffering from untreated addiction
and their loved ones. In addition, they have an outpatient program
and provide other recovery services.

Recovery Consultants, LLC (415) 306-7092

3020 Bridgeway #165, Sausalito, CA 94965. http://www.recovery-consultants.com. This consultancy provides one-to-one treatment and services to individuals & families struggle with substance abuse, mental and behavioral health disorders that extend beyond traditional treatment. Contact Shirley Wantland at shirley@recovery-consultants.com.

2

Family Recovery Coaches

NORTH BAY

Ron DeStefano, Ph.D. (415) 383-3489
342 Laverne Avenue, Mill Valley, CA 94941. Dr. DeStefano is a psychologist who works with families struggling with addiction. When appropriate, he integrates 12-step recovery and utilizes family systems therapy.

Full Circle Addiction & Recovery Services (415) 747-8224
775 Blithedale Avenue, Mill Valley, CA 94941. http://www. fullcirclerecoverycenter.net/intervention. This service, founded and facilitated by Kristina Wandzilak, endeavors to re-establish the connection between the family member suffering from untreated addiction and their loved ones. In addition, they have an outpatient program and provide intervention services.

Rosemary O'Connor, C.P.C. (415) 264-0078

189 Oak Drive, San Rafael, CA 94901. http://www.rocrecoveryservices.com. O'Connor, founder of ROC Recovery Services, is a Hazelden author, speaker and pioneer for mothers in recovery, and a life and addiction coach. She works in treatment placement for Hazelden Betty Ford.

Safe Passage Recovery (415) 578-2069

880 Las Gallians Avenue Suite 2, San Rafael, CA 94903. http://www.safepassagerecovery.com. This organization offers a family recovery program during a patient's 12-week individual outpatient program (IOP). This two-part intensive takes place at weeks six and twelve of the IOP. Each intensive explores the disease of addiction and its impact on the entire family via a multi-dimensional approach to learning and healing for individuals and their family system.

3

Addiction Physicians

SAN FRANCISCO

Paul Abramson, M.D. (415) 483-1528
450 Sutter Street Suite 840, San Francisco, CA 94108. http://www.
paulabramsonmd.com. Dr. Abramson is certified by the American
Board of Addiction Medicine. He specializes in the treatment of
chemical dependency and has special expertise in the use of bu-
prenorphine, baclofen, and benzodiazepine tapers. He also creates
customized IOP's.

NORTH BAY

David E. Smith, M.D. (415) 933-8759
854 Stanyan Street, San Francisco, CA 94117. Dr, Smith is an expert
on drugs, drug abuse and dependence. He is the founder of the
Haight Ashbery Free Clinic and the medical director of North Bay
Recovery Center, a men's dual diagnosis addiction treatment center.
He is also the medical director for Center Point drug rehabilitation
centers and Alta Mira recovery programs, among other positions.

Alex Zaphiris, M.D., M.S. (415) 388-2360
655 Redwood Highway #246, Mill Valley, CA 94941. http://www.360-md.com. support@360-MD.com. Dr. Zaphiris, of 360 MD, offers an integrative and addiction medical practice. He provides comprehensive care and whole-patient approach which integrates Western medicine and the best of evidence-based alternative medicine. He promotes personalized medical care which seeks to prevent and treat addiction.

The Second Edition of this Guide Will Be Released in Early 2018

If you are a health professional or program with expertise in helping patients and families with addiction, we would like to hear from you. To be included in the guide go to **www.merrittmentalhealth.com/addictionguide** and click on "Survey." You can also call (415) 285-3774 or email info@merrittmentalhealth.com.

4

Addiction-Informed Psychiatrists

SAN FRANCISCO

Eli Merritt, M.D. (415) 285-3774
3786 20th Street, San Francisco, CA 94100. http://www.merritt-mentalhealthcom. Dr. Merritt is the founder and director of Merritt Mental Health, a consulting and care navigation practice providing individualized guidance to patients and family members facing emotional crisis, relationship crisis, mental illness, or addiction. Merritt Mental Health helps patients and families find the best care possible to meet their needs in the Bay Area and beyond.

EAST BAY

Miran Choi, M.D. (510) 684-6834
2305 Ashby Avenue, Berkeley, CA 94705. http://www.mirancho-imd.com. choimd100@gmail.com. Dr. Choi offers general adult psychopharmacology and psychotherapy. She partners with clients to instill hope, manage cognitions, and develop new patterns. Her focus areas include anxiety, depression, ADHD, and PTSD.

PENINSULA

Carrie Griffin, M.D. (650) 315-7157
512 Hamilton Avenue, Palo Alto, CA 94301. carriegriffinmd@gmail.com. Dr. Griffin holds a private practice of general psychiatry for patients ages 16-65.

5

Other Addiction-Informed Physicians

SAN FRANCISCO

ReMeDy and SPARC Medical Groups (415) 651-4241
450 Post Street #900, San Francisco, CA 94102. http://www.remedydocs.com. ReMeDy is a multidisciplinary group of physicians who care for all musculoskeletal disorders. SPARCmed is a interdisciplinary medical group treating chronic pain and substance use disorders. These groups have locations both in San Francisco and the North Bay. Contact Mark J. Sontag, M.D. at marksontagmd@gmail.com.

Avril Swan, M.D. (415) 642-0333
1286 Sanchez Street, San Francisco, CA 94114. http://www.wholefamilymd.org. reception@wholefamilymd.org. Dr. Swan, of Whole Family MD, offers primary care for all ages.

6

Psychotherapists with Addiction Expertise

SAN FRANCISCO

Jeb Berkeley, Ph.D. (415) 563-8521
3405 Sacramento Street, San Francisco, CA 94118. http://www.jeberkeley.com. Dr. Berkeley's practice draws on mindfulness, EMDR, ACT, attachment theory, interpersonal neurobiology, family systems, and cognitive behavior therapies. He specializes in families and couples work.

Patt Denning, Ph.D. (415) 863-4282
45 Franklin Street Suite 320, San Francisco, CA 94102. http://www.harmreductiontherapy.org. Dr. Denning, of The Center for Harm Reduction Therapy, is one of the primary developers of harm reduction treatments for alcohol and other drug problems. She was named to the Drug Policy Resources Directory for the Media in the area of Dual Diagnosis and is a certified addiction specialist.

NORTH BAY

Matt Blagys (415) 849-2280
1191 Simmons Lane, Novato, CA 94945. http://www.livingatreflec-tions.com. Blagys is the clinical director at Reflections, an outpatient program. Reflections offers many different addiction therapy programs including dual diagnosis, holistic treatment, cognitive behavior, dialectical behavior, relapse prevention and family behavior therapies.

Ron DeStefano, Ph.D. (415) 383-3489
342 Laverne Avenue, Mill Valley, CA 94941. Dr. DeStefano is a psychologist who works with families struggling with addiction. When appropriate, he integrates 12-step recovery and utilizes family systems therapy.

Lilo Dixon, M.F.T. (415) 883-7652
342 Laverne Avenue, Mill Valley, CA 94941. Ms. Dixon is psychologist who focuses on evaluation, prevention, diagnosis, and treatment.

Jennifer Golick, Ph.D., L.M.F.T. 1-866-705-0828
1733 Skillman Lane, Petaluma, CA 94952 http://www.muirwood-teen.com. Dr. Golick is the Clinical Director at Muir Wood Adolescent and Family Services. Her specialties include cognitive behavior therapy and motivational interviewing, focusing on helping individuals and families identify problematic patterns of thinking in order to affect systemic change.

Marin City Wellness Center (415) 339-8813
630 Drake Avenue, Sausalito, CA 94965. http://www.marincityclinic.org. This center gathers a number of psychologists who provide therapy for those struggling with addiction. There is a licensed clinical social worker on site who provides case management services. This center accepts patients with MediCal and private insurance as well as offering a sliding scale.

Susan Montana, L.M.F.T. (707) 933-1469

793 1st Street West, Sonoma, CA 95476. Ms. Montana integrates cognitive behavior, dialectical behavior, and interpersonal therapies to address relationship difficulties and addictions. Ms. Montana is the clinical director of Safe Passage Recovery.

Wayne Thurston, Psy.D. 1-888-795-1965

11207 Valley Ford Road, Petaluma, CA 94952. http://www.olympiahouserehab.com. Dr. Thurston is a licensed clinical psychologist. He is the founder of Sonoma Recovery Services LLC and Olympia House. He has worked in addiction, mental health, and co-occurring disorders for nearly two decades.

EAST BAY

Katerina Melino, N.P. katerina@reveillerecovery.com

150 Moss Way, Oakland, CA 94611. http://www.reveillerecovery.com. Ms. Melino, of Reveille Recovery, offers supportive coaching for professionals seeking sobriety and maintaining recovery. In-person and web-based sessions are available.

PENINSULA

Stephanie Brown, Ph.D. (650) 322-0943

3445 Burgess Drive Suite 150, Menlo Park, CA 94025. http://www.stephaniebrownphd.com. info@stephaniebrownphd.com. Dr. Brown maintains a private practice and directs The Addictions Institute, an outpatient clinic. She also does therapist consultations and focuses on issues of trauma, including adult children of alcoholics with an emphasis on working within the developmental model of active addiction and recovery.

7

Residential Programs

SAN FRANCISCO

Henry Ohlhoff Men's Residential Program 1-877-677-4543
601 Steiner Street, San Francisco, CA 94117. http://www.ohlhoff. org/henry-ohlhoff-house. aprince@ohlhoff.org. This program is a long-term (6-12 months) 12-step treatment program for adult men with alcohol and drug dependency. It provides a structured, sober environment where men can focus on recovery while maintaining a regular work schedule, with treatment taking place on evenings and weekends.

Reflections (415) 234-4202
2253 Union Street #301, San Francisco, CA 94123. http://www. livingatreflections.com. This program provides dual diagnosis and co-occurring disorder residential treatment program. They offer a 30-to-90-day program. Therapists specialize in working with individuals suffering from trauma, unresolved grief and loss, addiction, and relapse.

Stepping Stone Women's Recovery Home (415) 751-5921
255 10th Avenue, San Francisco, CA 94118. http://www.stepping-stonehouse.org. info@steppingstonehouse.org. This program is a residential program designed specifically for working women in their early stages of recovery from alcoholism. Residents spend at least 32 hours per week in work, volunteer, or educational activities.

Walden House (415) 762-3705
Multiple locations in San Francisco. http://www.healthright360.org/agency/walden-house. This program is designed for those with substance use disorders, mental health issues, or co-occurring disorders. They work with high-risk populations from a variety of backgrounds, and accept the majority of participants as walk-ins, referrals from other agencies, and step-down transitional clients from residential treatment programs.

NORTH BAY

Alta Mira (415) 322-1350
125 Bulkley Avenue, Sausalito, CA. http://www.altamirarecovery.com. This center offers two programs. The 30-day program is designed for people who are in treatment for the first time, need a straightforward detox, and have no significant mental health issues. For those who have had treatment before, but were not able to maintain sobriety, their 90-day program is the best option.

Bayside Marin 1-877-434-0107
718 4th Street, San Rafael, CA 94901. http://www.baysidemarin.com/programs/residential/. This center offers inpatient drug treatment and the residential care for substance use and related disorders. Their facility is designed especially for guests who require privacy and exclusivity, as well as the latest in addiction and dual diagnosis treatment.

Five Sisters Ranch (707) 766-0755

1000 Longhorn Lane, Petaluma, CA 94952. http://www.fivesistersranch.com. This organization offers intensive programs for men and women. These programs provide cognitive and experiential tools for patients to explore and heal relational patterns. They specialize in helping clients maintain sobriety during relationship challenges.

Helen Vine Detox Center (415) 492-0818

301 Smith Ranch Road, San Rafael, CA 94903. This center offers mental health and substance abuse services. They provide residential short-term treatment (30 days or less). This is also a more affordable option for some patients, as they charge $200 per day.

Muir Wood Adolescent and Family Services 1-866-705-0828

1733 Skillman Lane, Petaluma, CA 94952. http://www.muirwoodteen.com. This center offers a comprehensive addiction and dual-diagnosis treatment program for boys. The typical length of stay is 45 to 90 days. For boys who are new to treatment and do not have significant behavioral or psychiatric issues, Muir Wood generally recommends a 45-day length of stay. For boys with a longer history of substance use or with significant behavioral or psychiatric issues, they recommend a stay of 60 to 90 days.

The Second Edition of this Guide Will Be Released in Early 2018

If you are a health professional or program with expertise in helping patients and families with addiction, we would like to hear from you. To be included in the guide go to **www.merrittmentalhealth.com/addictionguide** and click on "Survey." You can also call (415) 285-3774 or email info@merrittmentalhealth.com.

North Bay Recovery Center 1-844-249-9203
55 Shaver Street #200, San Rafael, CA 94901. http://www.north-bayrecoverycenter.com. This center offers addiction treatment for men. Their 90-day program includes group therapy sessions that focus on early recovery skills, relapse prevention skills, and social support in recovery. Individual counseling sessions may be scheduled to provide additional support or crisis management.

Olympia House 1-888-795-1965
11207 Valley Ford Road, Petaluma, CA 94954. http://www.olympiahouserehab.com. info@sonomarecoveryservices.com. info@sonomarecoveryservices.com. This program places focus on the active participation of the individual in developing a person-centered, individualized recovery plan. Treatment addresses the biological, psychological, social, and spiritual components of the individual while integrating the latests in evidence-based treatment. The average stay is 28 days.

PENINSULA

La Selva Group (650) 617-1759
206 South California Avenue, Palo Alto, CA 94306. http://www.thelaselvagroup.org. This organization provides individualized treatment and a comprehensive clinical program designed to help residents cope with the intrapsychic issues that interfere with an independent lifestyle. They provide a comfortable and safe alternative to inpatient psychiatric care.

NATIONAL

Back2Basics Outdoor Adventure Recovery 1-928-814-2220
1600 West University Avenue Suite 109, Flagstaff, AZ 86001. http://www.back2basicsoutdooradventures.com. This program offers six-month primary care for males ages 18-30. It consists of three days per week of outdoor adventure and four days per week of residential treatment. They offer an optional six-month transition program

as well as 12-step, individual, group therapy, and family workshops programs. Contact Roy DuPrez, M.Ed., at rduprez@b2badventures. com.

Breathe Life Healing Centers (415) 271-0132

8730 Sunset Boulevard, Suite 550, West Hollywood, California 90069. http://www.breathelifehealingcenters.com. This center offers a residential program treating drug and alcohol addiction, eating disorders, and co-occurring issues. They offer primary care, extended care, enhanced sober living, and outpatient services. Contact Dina Enberg, C.A.D.C. at dina.enberg@breathelhc.org.

Bridges to Recovery 1-888-997-2159

Los Angeles, CA. http://www.bridgestorecovery.com. This center has a core program of 30 to 60 days and a comprehensive program of 90 days, which offers continued work with a psychiatrist and clinical team, intensive workshops for families, and adaptive living programming to support reintegrating after rehabilitation.

Burning Tree Ranch 1-972-997-2159

2837 County Road #101, Kaufman, TX 75142. http://www.burning-tree.com. This program offers a long-term inpatient program which promotes an innovative curriculum based on holistic treatment and spiritual principles that treat the whole person. They also incorporate proven medical and mental health interventions.

Hazelden Betty Ford 1-503-554-4300

1901 Esther Street, Newberg, OR 97132. http://www.hazeldenbetty-ford.org. This organization provides a number of treatments in slightly different structures and intensities, but an abstinence-based, 12-step approach utilizing evidence-based practices are core to all programs. Core treatment activities include individual therapy, educational lectures, group therapy, and special-focus groups. Their Springbrook campus in Newberg, Oregon is also recognized for addiction treatment for patients who have a history of trauma and medication-assisted opioid addiction treatment.

Northbound 1-866-311-0003
4343 Von Karman Avenue #100, Newport Beach, CA 92660. http://www.livingsober.com. This center has separate men's and women's residential programs, which both emphasize holistic therapies, evidence-based treatment, experiential opportunities, 12-step processes, and educational groups. LINKS Christian-based programming is available for those interested in implementing Christianity in their recovery.

The Ranch 1-931-219-1819
6107 Pinewood Road, Nunnelly, TN 37137. https://www.recovery-ranch.com. This facility specializes in attachment disorder and utilizes many different therapies to support patients during their treatment.

Spring Lake Ranch 1-802-492-3322
1169 Spring Lake Road, Cuttingsville, VT 05738. http://www.spring-lakeranch.org. This program provides a work-centered therapy community. Working on a diverse Vermont farm is combined with regular sessions with on-site therapists.

Willingway Hospital 1-888-979-2140
311 Jones Mill Road, Statesboro, GA 30458. http://www.willingway.com. This hospital has separate facilities for men and women, including a long-term treatment program which usually lasts for one year. The program is structured to focus on emotional stabilization, education about the illness of addiction, development of recovery resources and skills, and personal adoption of recovery principles.

8

Outpatient Programs

SAN FRANCISCO

Bayside Marin 1-877-434-0107
Financial District. San Francisco, CA. http://www.baysidemarin.com/programs/outpatient/. This addiction rehab center offers a comprehensive outpatient program that meets three-to-four days per week, either mornings or evenings, in order to accommodate the patients schedule. The program's features include individualized treatment panning, acupuncture, yoga and meditation, referral to self-help support groups, and Lifelong Continuing Care. This program is also available in San Rafael.

Foundations San Francisco (415) 293-1680
55 Francisco Street Suite 405, San Francisco, CA 94113. http://www.foundationsrecoverynetwork.com. This program offers comprehensive outpatient treatment. Flexible daytime and evening programs address addiction and any co-occuring mental health issues simultaneously.

Walden House (415) 762-3705

Multiple locations in San Francisco. http://www.healthright360. org/agency/walden-house. This program is designed for those with substance use disorders, mental health issues, or co-occurring disorders. Walden House works with high-risk populations from a variety of backgrounds, and accepts the majority of participants, including walk-in's, referrals from other agencies and step-down transitional clients from residential treatment programs.

NORTH BAY

Alta Mira 1-877-978-1805

591 Redwood Highway #5220, Mill Valley, CA 94941. http://www. altamirarecovery.com. This center's 8-week program is founded on evidence-based treatment methods, including mindfulness-based relapse prevention, cognitive behavior, and dialectical behavior therapies.

Bayside Marin 1-877-434-0107

718 4th Street, San Rafael, CA 94901. http://www.baysidemarin. com/programs/outpatient/. This addiction rehab center offers a comprehensive outpatient program meets three-to-four days per week, either mornings or evenings, in order to accommodate the patients schedule. The program's features include individualized treatment panning, acupuncture, yoga and meditation, referral to self-help support groups, and Lifelong Continuing Care. This program is also available in San Francisco's financial district.

Center Point DAAC (707) 544-3295

2403 Professional Drive, Santa Rosa, CA 9540. http://www.daacinfo.org. This program provides individual, family, and group counseling with bilingual options. The length of treatment is based on an individual's needs and completion of individualized treatment goals. Family members are encouraged to participate in the program.

Full Circle Addiction & Recovery Services (415) 747-8224
775 Blithedale Avenue, Mill Valley, CA 94941. http://www.full-circlerecoverycenter.net/intervention. This organization offers a 10-week IOP program, which includes 9 hours per week of educational and therapeutic process groups and weekly individual therapy sessions. Their program provides clinical treatment for those struggling with chemical dependence, while maintaining or building their active lives.

Muir Wood Adolescent and Family Services (415) 785-8724
938 B Street, San Rafael, CA 94901. http://www.muirwoodteen.com. This organization's outpatient program serves both adolescent males and females ages 12-19 with substance use disorder and co-occurring behavioral health issues. Their team works closely with teens and families to develop an individualized treatment plan that may include group, cognitive behavior, and dialectal behavior therapies as well as medication management and neuropsychological testing on a case-by-case basis.

Olympia House 1-888-795-1965
11207 Valley Ford Road, Petaluma, CA 94954. http://www.olympiahouserehab.com. info@sonomarecoveryservices.com. This program places focus on the active participation of the individual in developing a person-centered, individualized recovery plan. Treatment addresses the biological, psychological, social, and spiritual components of the individual while integrating evidence-based treatment.

Reflections (415) 849-2287
770 Tamalpais Drive #206, Corte Madera, CA 94925. http://www.livingatreflections.com. This center offers an outpatient program that lasts an average of 12 weeks, with group and individual services lasting 10 to 12 hours per week. The treatment program consists of two individual therapy sessions per week coupled with multiple group therapy sessions and educational didactic groups.

Safe Passage Recovery (415) 578-2069
880 Las Gallians Avenue Suite 2, San Rafael, CA 94903. http://www.safepassagerecovery.com. This organization offers a 12-week program that centers on the Identity Transformation Model which facilitates full reintegration into a sober life for clients. Safe Passage utilizes a biopsychosocial-model focus in treatment, which attributes addiction to biological, psychological, and social factors. Spirituality is another component in treatment.

PENINSULA

La Selva Group (650) 617-1759
206 South California Avenue, Palo Alto, CA 94306. http://www.thelaselvagroup.org. This organization offers an outpatient services program to empower clients to reach their maximum level of functioning and live more fulfilled lives. They also offer residential services.

NATIONAL

Northbound 1-866-311-0003
4343 Von Karman Avenue #100, Newport Beach, CA 92660. http://www.livingsober.com. This center's outpatient program is most appropriate for those living in Orange County and working during the day. The program includes 12-step meetings, group therapy sessions, daily check-ins with a case manager, court services, alcohol and drug testing, and individualized treatment plans.

9

Medical Detox

SAN FRANCISCO

Walden House (415) 762-3705
Multiple locations in San Francisco. http://www.healthright360.org/agency/walden-house. This organization's Social Detox Center is a 3-to-7 day detoxification program. Length of stay is determined by a variety of factors, including the history and severity of addiction and need for ongoing stabilization services.

NORTH BAY

Aurora Hospital (707) 800-770
1287 Fulton Road, Santa Rosa, CA 95401. http://www.aurorasantarosa.com. This hospital helps patients detox with a psychiatric-based approach.

Bayside Marin 1-877-434-0107
718 4th Street, San Rafael, CA 94901. http://www.baysidemarin.com/programs/detox/. This addiction rehab center offers detoxification in a safe, non-hospital residential home setting. In addition

to their residential detoxification program, Bayside offers a 7-day, detoxification-only program. From this 7-day detoxification, patients may enter their residential program or their intensive outpatient program.

Helen Vine Detox Center (415) 492-0818
301 Smith Ranch Road, San Rafael, CA 94903. This center offers mental health and substance use services. They provide residential, short-term treatment (30 days or less). It is also a more affordable option for some patients, as they charge $200 a day.

Howard Kornfeld, M.D. and Associates (415) 383-2949
3 Madrona Street, Mill Valley, CA 94941. http://www.recovery-withoutwalls.com. drkornfeld@gmail.com. Dr. Kornfeld and his associates work with addiction and pain medicine. This is an evidence-based medical practice that joins psychotherapy, detoxification, medication, addiction counseling, nutritional guidance, and mindfulness.

Marin General Hospital (415) 925-7663
250 Bon Air Road, Greenbrae, CA 94904. http://www.detoxrehabs.org/center/marin-general-hospital. This hospital offers medical detox.

EAST BAY

John Muir Hospital (925) 674-4114
2740 Grant Street, Concord, CA 94520. This hospital provides detoxification and treatment for alcohol and substance abuse. Their team of specialized doctors and nurses supervises patients' safe withdrawal. During this process, patients participate in an educational and therapeutic treatment process until they are medically stabilized.

PENINSULA

Mills Peninsula Medical Center (650) 696-4666
100 South San Mateo Drive, San Mateo, CA 94401. http://www.mills-peninsula.org/behavioral-health/substance-abuse-treatment/acute-detoxification.html. This organization's substance abuse treatment center provides intensive medical management of acute detoxification for adults age 18 and older in a confidential hospital unit.

NATIONAL

Hazelden Betty Ford 1-503-554-4300
1901 Esther Street, Newberg, OR 97132. http://www.hazeldenbettyford.org. This this organization's detox program is supervised by medical staff who may use medications to reduce the discomfort of withdrawal. Every patient admitted to inpatient program must go through 24-hour detox. Their Springbrook campus in Newberg, Oregon is also recognized for addiction treatment for patients who have a history of trauma and medication-assisted opioid addiction treatment.

Northbound 1-866-311-0003
4343 Von Karman Avenue #100, Newport Beach, CA 92660. http://www.livingsober.com. This fully licensed, sub-acute residential detox center provides a safe, supervised environment in addition to therapeutic services. Detox is overseen by Medical Director Dr. Edward Kaufman, former president of the American Academy of Addiction Psychiatry.

Las Vegas Recovery Center 1-800-790-0091
3371 North Buffalo Drive, Las Vegas, NV 89129. http://lasvegasrecovery.com. This program offers individualized detox treatment which closely monitors the individual with special attention to rest,

nutrition and fluid replacement. Protocols can include a variety of medications when appropriate and necessary. Dr. Mel Pohl is the Chief Medical Officer at this center.

Willingway Hospital 1-888-979-2140
311 Jones Mill Road, Statesboro, GA 30458. http://www.willingway. com. This hospital offers a detox program run by addiction medicine physicians, making it ideal for complicated cases such as high level methadone addiction and other difficult detoxifications. Detoxification usually precedes inpatient treatment.

10

Child & Adolescent Resources

NORTH BAY

Center Point DAAC (707) 544-3295
2403 Professional Drive, Santa Rosa, CA 9540. http://www.daacinfo.org. This program provides outpatient treatment for youth ages 12-18 in which family members are encouraged to participate. Because most youth qualify for MediCal, treatment can be free. There is also an Alternatives to Detention program serving youth ages 14-17 who are at risk or currently in referral from County Juvenile Probation.

Muir Wood Adolescent and Family Services IOP (415) 785-8724
938 B Street, San Rafael, CA 94901. http://www.muirwoodteen. com. This organization's outpatient program serves both adolescent males and females ages 12-19 with substance use disorder and co-occurring behavioral health issues. Their team works closely with teens and families to develop an individualized treatment plan that may include group, cognitive behavior, and dialectal behavior therapies as well as medication management and neuropsychological testing on a case-by-case basis.

Muir Wood Adolescent and Family Services
Residential Program 1-866-705-0828

1733 Skillman Lane, Petaluma, CA 94952. http://www.muirwood-teen.com. This center offers a comprehensive addiction and dual-diagnosis treatment program for boys. The typical length of stay is 45 to 90 days. For boys who are new to treatment and do not have significant behavioral or psychiatric issues, they generally recommend a 45-day length of stay. For boys with a longer history of substance use, or with significant behavioral or psychiatric issues, they recommend a stay of 60 to 90 days.

CALIFORNIA

Betty Ford Family & Children's Center 1-866-280-8564

Locations in Los Angeles, Riverside County, San Diego and elsewhere in California. http://www.www.hazeldenbettyford.org/treatment/family-children/childrens-program. This program is for children ages 7-12 who need to stay healthy and safe when their parent is suffering from addiction. The 3-or-4-day sessions teach kids about addiction through age-appropriate activities.

Bill Lane & Associates Adolescent Transport Services
1-866-492-3400

http://www.billlaneandassociates.com. This organization's goal is to alleviate parental anxieties, move children safely and efficiently to appropriate resources and, in the process, help everyone make a smooth transition to the potentially lifesaving opportunity that treatment provides.

11

Sober Living

SAN FRANCISCO

Reflections (415) 234-4202
2253 Union Street #301, San Francisco, CA 94123. www.livingatreflections.com. This center offers an eight-week, dual diagnosis drug and alcohol treatment program focused on providing individuals with comprehensive treatment for substance abuse. The center also provides life and self-care skills to ensure a smooth transition back to mainstream life.

Walden House (415) 762-3705
Multiple locations in San Francisco. http://www.healthright360. org/agency/walden-house. This organization's Sober Living Environment Program is an interim step-down level of care for participants who have achieved significant progress toward treatment goals, but who are not yet ready to fully step down to community-based living. Individuals may live in this transitional environment for up to one year.

NORTH BAY

Safe Passage Recovery, Golden Gate House (415) 578-2069
880 Las Gallians Avenue Suite 2, San Rafael, CA 94903. http://www.safepassagerecovery.com. This organization offers a CCAPP-certified sober living environment in Tiburon, CA. Their emphasis is on providing structure, accountability, and stability within a safe and sober environment. It provides residents with the space to heal and thrive as they transition to life in recovery.

CALIFORNIA

Safe Harbor Treatment Centers for Women 1-949-645-1026
240 Knox Street, Costa Mesa, CA 92627. http://www.safeharborhouse.com This center's 90-day program takes place in a homes nestled in a residential neighborhood. Women in this program experience real-life scenarios and utilize the wisdom they have previously gained at an inpatient program. The program offers education and treatment for co-occurring eating disorders and codependency. It utilizes a 12-step program philosophy.

The Second Edition of this Guide Will Be Released in Early 2018

If you are a health professional or program with expertise in helping patients and families with addiction, we would like to hear from you. To be included in the guide go to **www.merrittmentalhealth.com/addictionguide** and click on "Survey." You can also call (415) 285-3774 or email info@merrittmentalhealth.com.

12

Educational Consultants

EAST BAY

Shayna Abraham, M.A. (650) 888-4575
Prepare To Bloom, LLC. P.O. Box 31520 Walnut Creek CA 94565.
http://www.preparetobloom.com.   shayna@preparetobloom.com.
Ms. Abraham offers therapeutic and educational consulting services for children, adolescents, and young adults.

13

Books Related to Addiction Treatment

The End of My Addiction
Olivier Ameisen, M.D.
This book is both a memoir of Dr. Ameisen's own struggle and a call to action for research that can rescue millions from the scourge of addiction and spare their loved ones from the damage of the disease. It chronicles how the author experimented with the muscle relaxer baclofen to free himself from the craving for alcohol.

Unchain Your Brain:
10 Steps to Breaking the Addictions that Steal Your Life
Daniel G. Amen, M.D. and David E. Smith, M.D.
This books offers a practical, step-by-step program that shows readers how to boost their brain so they can kick bad habits. It provides information on how to get the right evaluation to ensure that readers or their loved ones can heal from addition, strategies for boosting one's brain to get control of addiction, and more.

A Sober Mom's Guide to Recovery:
Taking Care of Yourself to Take Care of Your Kids
Rosemary O'Connor

At once affirming, engaging, and practical, this book combines down-to-earth advice with the inspiring stories of recovering mothers, including the author's, to offer guidance on over fifty topics including stress, relapse, relationships, sex and intimacy, spirituality, shame, gratitude, dating, and parenting. This book draws from the author's many years of experience working with women in recovery.

The Lost Years:
Surviving a Mother and Daughter's Worst Nightmare
Kristina Wandzilak and Constance Curry

This book is the real life story of a child struggling with alcohol and drug addiction and a mother unable to save her. Each offers a first-hand account of the years lost to addiction and despair as well as a story of recovery. The book discusses co-dependency and offers perspective to families with a family member suffering from addiction.

Previous title by Dr. Eli Merritt

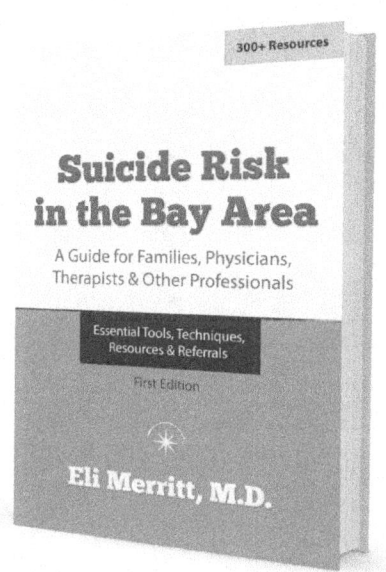

Suicide Risk in the Bay Area: A Guide for Families, Physicians, Therapists, and Other Professionals combines a suicide prevention resource directory, containing over 300 local resources, with a step-by-step guide on how to assess, manage, and talk about suicide risk.

Throughout the book, the message is clear: Talk About It. The Introduction offers lessons from Dr. Merritt's psychiatric practice, followed by more than fifty educational modules providing vignettes, tips and checklists to help readers to talk about suicide risk effectively and compassionately. At the same time, the directory collects hotlines, mobile crisis units, suicide prevention trainings, and other crucial resources from the four major regions of the Bay Area.

In the book's Foreword, Renée Binder, M.D., President of the American Psychiatric Association, offes that *Suicide Risk in the Bay Area* "deserves to be on the desk of every mental health professional who lives and works in the Bay Area."

To order a copy, just search for "Suicide Risk in the Bay Area" on Amazon.com.